EVERYDAY

with M:

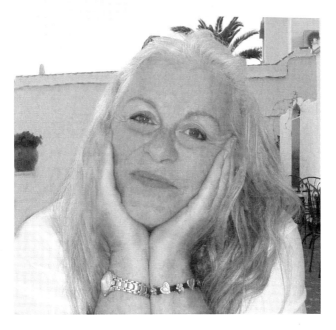

There is so much information available today on improving your vitality, stamina, health, happiness and energy flows that it is easy to become confused, overwhelmed and end up doing absolutely nothing!

Let Madison guide you through what she considers to be the real 'key players' in the energy medicine arena, the techniques that deliver consistent results that really work.

Use this book as a blueprint for formulating a daily energy routine, unique to you, that you can use for the rest of your life.

First published in Great Britain

All paper used in the printing of this book has been made from wood grown in managed, sustainable forests.

ISBN13: 978-1-78003-511-6

Essential Book Series

First published by Indepenpress Publishing Limited

25 Eastern Place

Brighton

BN2 1GJ

For Author Essentials

A catalogue record of this book is available from

the British Library

Cover design © Author Essentials

info@authoressentials.com

It is all about *creating space* for energy to flow, this is our mantra throughout the whole book!

The only props you will need are:

- Yoga belt for stretching, or improvise with a scarf

- Cheap, spiked plastic hairbrush

- A throw or mat for the floor work

- Optional – incense stick/gentle music

- Ideal – do outside in Nature

LISTEN TO YOURSELF

I would encourage you to take 30 seconds or so of quiet time to scan your body before and after the exercises – how do you feel? Where is there a block, pain, tightness, stiffness? Tune in to yourself, you are the very best judge of what is going on in you and therefore what you need to feel better in both a physical and emotional sense.

The first section is a small core of exercises that are 'non-negotiable'; you have to do them every day! These provide you with a firm foundation stone upon which everything else is built, it is the nucleus from which you bloom.

The second section [Maddie's Pick 'n Mix] honours our unique individuality, there are 31 exercises featured, try a different one each day, take time to listen, to tune in and objectively evaluate how it feels: does it feel good? Does it feel as if it is doing something? If the answers are yes then consider adding it to your daily routine, if the answers are no, then put it in your personal recycle bin to pull out another day, another time when it might be more relevant.

You can't do everything. Focus on being discerning and selecting those techniques that really suit your body at this moment in time. Take a month to refine your daily routine with clarity and precision so that you get the maximum benefit with the minimum of effort.

Most of all *enjoy* compiling your personalised energy programme – it has to be fun, it has to feel good or, unless you are the strictest of disciplinarians and have willpower like Madonna – you will not stick to it and it will fade away as other ideas have done in the past. Far better to do a couple of exercises every day than nothing and once you begin to feel the benefits you will be more motivated to keep up your practice and build a stable daily energy 'habit'.

The third section features a few little energy tips I have picked up along the way.

> *"By stimulating the flow of energy, the body's own healing network can be activated."*

Roger Callahan, Ph.D., Tapping the Healer Within.

As always, I would ask you to be sensible and if you are suffering any aches, pains, stiffness or under doctor's orders, please check with your healthcare practitioner before attempting any exercise routine, just to be safe.

EVERYDAY ENERGY – CONTENTS

THE NON NEGOTIABLES – *3 minutes, at a time convenient to YOU*

MADDIE'S PICK 'N MIX

"The higher your structure is to be, the deeper must be its foundations"

[Saint Augstine 396-430]

In Energy Medicine, you assess where the energy system needs attention and correct the energy disturbances. Energy medicine is both a complement to other systems of medical care and, in itself, a complete system for self-care and self-help. It can address physical illness and emotional disorders, and it can also promote wellness and peak performance. There are myriad energy disturbances and a vast array of techniques to correct them. However, *the exercises in this book represent the most common disturbances that show up time and time again on most people.* They are to do with our foundation flows, the core of our energy integrity.

Doing them will ensure your energies are running in the right direction along their pathways, crossing in the right way, hooked up to each other – *you will be returning them to default mode!*

"Energy pathways" referred to as *meridians* in traditional Chinese medicine are also described in a variety of other healing traditions. We live in exciting times, where science is beginning to prove the existence of energy in its many forms. A study published in the *Proceedings of the National Academy of Science* in 1998 using functional Magnetic Resonance Imaging (MRI) demonstrated that stimulating an acupuncture point in the toe (each acupuncture point is believed to sit on the line of and regulate the energy in a particular meridian) activated the

1

exact areas of the brain that would be predicted by acupuncture theory, despite no known anatomical pathways connecting the toe to that brain region. A special camera shows that when stimulated, the meridians generate light along channels that are identical to the descriptions of meridians found in the texts of traditional Chinese medicine. The meridians and corresponding acupuncture points also exhibit other physical characteristics such as less electromagnetic resistance, enhanced ultrasound attenuation, and the conduction of light, infrared, and microwaves.

Follow your instinct and if something just doesn't 'feel right' then omit it, or adapt it so that it feels good to you... you will KNOW when it is right for you!

Be flexible in your interpretation of the guidelines, if you feel like doing an exercise in a slightly different way, or for longer or shorter than the recommended time – then do it your way.

*Your Inner Sage will know better than me, what **your** body needs.*

In summary, these exercises will...

- Begin to balance every system of your body, building immunity, increasing its ability to process foods and life itself.

- Retain flexibility in body, mind and energy.

- Allow you to dismantle energetic and emotional obstacles and move forward in your life.

- Support, in fact sometimes enhance, any therapist treatments you are receiving.

- Support and help you cope with side effects of any medical intervention or surgery you may be receiving.

- Lift your mood and rekindle optimism.

- Encourage optimum Strangeflow function – these extraordinary ancient flows of energy, are primarily 'trouble shooters' for your entire body, help return joy to your life and deal with change.

- Help you focus and concentrate.

- Increase your vitality and stamina.

- Achieve well-being on all levels.

- Energy flow freely, thus preventing/easing disease and pain.

- Release your 'Inner Healer' to cope more effectively with physical challenges in life.

- Lift you out of that 'spiritual armchair'.

To be frank, it is pointless to move on to more complicated energy techniques, if your foundations aren't strong; the corrections just will not hold.

As humans we tend to have an insatiable urge to move onwards and upwards to the complex and complicated, sometimes running before we have really mastered walking. So, I would urge you to take this opportunity to intuitively mould your own personal foundation energy stone. Once that is strong, as Saint Augstine said: you can build it high!

Make a pact that you will have patience and faithfully road test the daily routine and each technique over the next month, at the end of which *you* choose *your* favourites to make up your very own daily practice and then DO IT for six weeks and FEEL the difference it makes to you on all levels.

This is the beginning of your personalised energy 'toolbox'!

SOME REMINDERS

1. BREATHING is important – at no time should you hold your breath. This sounds so obvious, but it is remarkable, how many people will stop breathing when they concentrate on an exercise.

2. As a rule of thumb, on movement/effort, breathe OUT and let the **abdominal girdle** do the work [for example when you come out of a forward bend]. This will help prevent back strain.

3. Never at any time do a movement that causes you physical pain. That is the body's way of warning you to stop. Obey it.

4. Energy flows were attention goes, so keep your **attention and intention** focussed sharply on what you are doing. If you are restricted physically, just imag-

ining your body doing these exercises will have a beneficial effect.[1]

5. Let go of your worries and anxieties and focus on how your body feels. **Reconnect** with it. Observe how it reacts.

6. Any other thoughts should be of self-love, gratitude, and forgiveness, in short – the *positive* emotions of life. Don't do these exercises contemplating what you are going to serve up to the kids for dinner tonight!

7. Don't be an exercise martyr. Change your attitude and start viewing the time allocated to your exercise routine as one of **life's** *treats*, not punishment. Think of this as precious time for *you.* If you have space, create a special corner in your house or garden just for you.

8. Don't become an **'Energy Bore'** – yes, it is good to share things with friends but not to any extreme. If your enthusiasm is received with glazed eyes, back off, not everyone is ready or willing to work with their energies. Some people can be positively rude about anything outside their comfort zone, so why put yourself in a situation where you are under attack. Energy work is not for everyone, or should I say not everyone is ready for energy work; so respect some peoples' rejection of it.

---

1 In his book WHY ZEBRAS DON'T GET ULCERS, Robert M Sapolsky cites the work of neurologist Antonio Damasio: a study was done on the conductor Herbert von Karajan, showing that the maestro's heart would race just as wildly when he was listening to a piece of music as when he was conducting it. Thoughts can evoke powerful physical reactions in the body, so use this to your advantage – THINK exercise!

Sometimes there is **wisdom in silence.** This took me some time to learn, as I had an almost evangelical enthusiasm about energy work and wanted to heal the entire world. Just call me Pollyanna. Nowadays I am much more laid back and do not impose my views on anyone. On the other hand, if someone asks, well, the floodgates do tend to open! The information is there and it is your choice if you pick it up or not, but by the sheer fact you are reading this, I suspect you are open minded!

9. **Prepare** – choose a quiet place and read in detail what you will be doing and then do it! At first it will take you longer as you will be constantly referring to the book, but after a while, once you know the routine and can put the book away, it will take less time.

10. My DVD[2] features a Daily Energy Exercise section. There are also clips on You Tube – just tap in Madison food testing and voila! There I am. You can also visit my site: www.midlifegoddess.ning.com and click on the video section.

11. Don't restrict yourself to set times. If you suddenly feel like doing a particular exercise – DO IT – your body is signalling that it needs it. The more you work with your energies, the more sensitive you become to your body's needs – you will begin to sense it's requirements as and when they arise and how to meet those needs.

12. **Create the time** to do them – get up earlier, watch less television – whatever it takes, plan when and where you will do them. The ideal setting is on a

2 Copies can be ordered via www.midlifegoddess.ning.com

beach, a cliff top, on grass, in a forest. i.e. out in Nature. However even if a tiny urban 'bed-sit' is your environment, they will still work!

13. Decide on your **time commitment** and enter it in your diary – book out the time. The Virgos among you will find this appealing! In this way you can plan around your workouts and are in no danger of 'forgetting' to do them.

14. If you have time, create a **sympathetic environment**, light a candle, turn off the phone, burn incense[3] and make a real ritual out of your workout. Rituals tend to focus the attention thus improving effectiveness.

15. Alternatively associate an **everyday activity** with a particular exercise. For example, do a Cross Crawl every time you wait for the kettle to boil, Trace Regulator flow when you get out of the shower, Four Thumps when you clean your teeth. Make use of 'post it' notes to remind you.

16. **SMILE…** it is the simplest Energy Exercise and will enhance any work you do.

"If a warrior is to succeed at anything, the success must come gently,

with a great deal of effort but

with no stress or obsession."

Carlos Castaneda

---

3 Incense is highly personal, try Nag Champra or Nag Champra Satya, two of my favourites

So my energy warriors, the bottom line is:

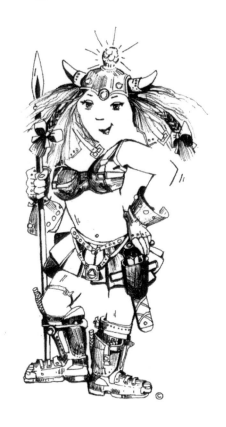

Thank you to Salli Young for my mini energy warrior

It does take effort; they will not work unless you do them on a regular basis. However, after a while a habit forms and they will cease to be a chore and become a daily joy.

Every aspect of your life will benefit from returning harmony to your flows.

Don't be an energy 'snob', rushing to the most advanced techniques and ignoring the simple fundamentals; *enjoy the humble joy of working with your foundations so that you don't build your house on clay.*

WHY should you do any of the energy workouts?

There are a number of very good reasons, they help:

- retain flexibility in body, mind and energy

- allow you to remove energetic obstacles and move forward in your life

- support any therapist treatments you are receiving

- lift your mood

- increase your vitality and joy in life

- achieve well-being on all levels

- energy flow freely, thus preventing disease and pain

- release your 'Inner Healer' to cope more effectively with physical challenges in life

- reduce the effects of stress on the body – bear in mind that 99.9999% of all physical problems we have are caused or exacerbated by stress.

- to simply feel better and enjoy your life to the full – whatever age you are.

Lastly – don't forget to smile, the simplest energy exercise in the world.

THE NON NEGOTIABLES – *these are the nucleus of your routine*

The 4 THUMPS

just 5 seconds each one

I have been talking a lot about 'energy', what exactly do I mean?

Energy is a life-force that flows through and around our bodies. It is the blueprint, the infrastructure, the invisible foundation for the health of your body.

"Curtis and Hurtak propose, the meridian system may be a distinct energy system that "functions alongside the accepted blood circulatory, lymphatic, and nervous systems," capable of reading, coding, and transmitting information from one part of the body to another and providing "an underlying template for the physical body. They believe it operates on a distinct energetic spectrum whose movement is more like an energy wave than a tube or vessel. Supporting the hypothesis that this energy system impacts biological processes, abundant anecdotal and limited empirical evidence suggests that disruption in a meridian pathway precedes (and, again, thus predicts) disease in specific organs served by that meridian, and that meridians whose energies are disrupted can be treated for therapeutic benefit." [quote from David Feinstein – Energy Psychology][4]

It is not a figment of an overactive bohemian imagination but can be clearly measured by scientific equipment

---

4 www.innersource.net

[e.g. MRI or EEG] and captured by Kirlian photography. Fascinating research is taking place right now regarding the harnessing of the 'energy' of thought, to a prosthetic limb to control its movement.

Like radio, TV, cell phone waves, the wind and electricity, energy cannot be seen with the naked eye, but it is most definitely there.

It exists and without it, we would not.

The foundation stone of good health is a free flowing energy system. There are many different types of energy 'medicine' practices, but all ultimately deal with finding a balance.

If the 'flow' is disturbed in any way, due to stress or trauma it has repercussions on the physical body: lowered immunity, increased food intolerances, increased vulnerability to infections, diminished ability to cope with the challenges of life, fatigue, lethargy, depression, lack of efficiency of the major organs and systems – it hits every single part of your body. The effects may be subtle at first but cumulative and over years can contribute to ill health.

There are different energy systems in the body that work in pure synergy. As you get to know your energies and more importantly energy disruptions and how to correct them, you can often prevent physical symptoms manifesting.

The body has remarkable self-healing powers but these can only achieve their full potential if the energies are balanced and free flowing. So, to release your 'Inner Healer', start paying attention to your flows!

There are 'meridians' of energy running through the body, think of them as motorways connecting the different organs and systems. Energy should run in a specific direction along each channel. However, due to stress, physical or emotional exhaustion or trauma, energy can sometimes *'flip into reverse'* and literally run backwards along the meridians, going the wrong way up that motorway and causing chaos.

If this happens you may:

- lack focus/concentration/clarity of thought,
- feel tired,
- possibly be depressed most of the time and life can seem as if you are pushing water uphill,
- Your immunity will be compromised resulting in frequent, niggling coughs and colds.
- None of your systems will operate to full potential
- Never feel 100% well

If that sounds familiar, maybe your energies are 'reversed'.

Get back in the right lane, flip your energies back into the correct direction with the following technique [the 4 thumps], it takes all of 20 seconds. Do it 5-6 times a day and see if you feel better and life seems a bit easier.

Form your thumb and first two fingers into a triad and firmly massage or tap the points described below.

If you have long nails, simply improvise and use your knuckles. Don't forget to breath and smile while you tap.

The benefits of this simple exercise include:–

- 'Flips' energy into forward flow.

- Jump-starts and energises the entire system.

- Balances disruptions caused by travelling, especially through time zones. [A great one to do during a flight and when you step off the plane].

- Brings clarity to thought.

- Improves focus and concentration.

- Brings a flow back into your life.

- Temporarily energises the eyes, useful if you are tired but still have a few more miles to drive.

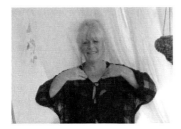 You will be tapping and therefore stimulating the 27th acupuncture point on each Kidney meridian. These important points act as 'junction boxes' for other meridians.

They are located near the 'right angle' where the collar and breast bones meet. You will feel two natural indentations that may be slightly tender when you press them.

Don't worry if you can't find the exact points, you know the approximate area, so tap around and you will get them, as with all energy work, it is about intention and attention.

Breathe, fully moving your rib cage and diaphragm.

Smile and tap for 5 seconds.

Benefits of this second thump include:

- Stimulates the Thymus gland.

- Supports the Immune System.

- Helps cope with the body's stress response and negative emotional energies.

- Stimulates overall energy and vitality – primates will thump this gland to increase their strength before mating or fighting.

- Places the body in a temporary state of 'balance'.

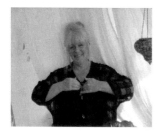
You will be tapping over the Thymus Gland[5] which is located in the middle of your chest – exactly where Tarzan thumps, in fact rather than tapping; you could clench your fists and thump your chest like Tarzan!

Breathe, smile and tap/thump for 5 seconds.

The monkey thump

– Benefits of monkey thumping include:

- Boosts Immune System and general energy levels.

---

5 The Australian psychiatrist, Dr John Diamond [Your Body Doesn't Lie] www.drjohndiamond.com – made a study of the Thymus gland and suggests we 'waltz' the thymus, i.e. tap lightly to the waltz rhythm... 123 123 123, smile and look at something beautiful while you are tapping to increase the effectiveness of the exercise.

14

- Increases your ability to accept/metabolise changes.

- Balances blood chemistry.

- Aids detoxification of the body.

- Helps metabolise and absorb nutrients.

- Improves absorption of supplements [tap for a few seconds before and after taking them].

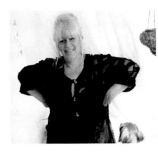 You will be massaging/tapping/thumping the 21st acupressure points on each Spleen meridian. These are located on the side of the ribcage, roughly where the bottom line of a bra would sit [see photo]. You will know when you hit on them as they will be tender.

Once located, use your clenched fists to massage, tap or thump firmly the points for a minimum of 5 seconds. Breathe and smile.

You can also work on the Spleen lymphatic points: simply lean back slightly, opening up the ribcage and tap round from Sp21 to underneath each breast in line with the nipples.

Cheeky thump

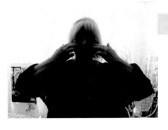

- Relieves anxiety

- Helps you begin to trust in the mystery of life

- Helps in letting issues

pass through, be digested and released

- Balanced Stomach energy encourages you to pay attention to self-care
- Helps achieve a clear thought process.

Called the 'Great Bone Hole' they are located slightly below the apex of your cheeks when you smile, in line with your eye and the edge of your nostril.

Again, do for 5 seconds.

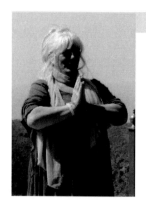

Thymus pressure with prayer

Place your palms together in a prayer position. Forearms parallel with the floor. Thumbs will be over the Thymus gland, push against this point firmly for ten seconds then release. Repeat. This brings you into a temporary state of balance and in the ancient Indian tradition, connects you to your soul.

Say a simple thank you for all your blessings.

Start cultivating an attitude of humility and gratitude.

Cross crawl – 20 seconds

- Do you feel tired for no real reason?
- Do you have a tendency to pessimism or depression?

- Are you slowly becoming a lethargic sloth?

- Is motivating yourself to do anything a major task?

- Do you find your memory is not what it was?

- Do you lack clarity and focus in your thinking?

- Rather than feel energised by exercise does it tend to tire you?

- Do you feel you are only operating at about 50% efficiency?

- Are you constantly getting niggling coughs and colds?

- Do you feel that your senses are less acute?

If the answer is 'yes' to any of the above, read on. The Cross Crawl could definitely be of help to you.

The body functions with crossing patterns, curves, roundness and above all, flow. There are very few sharp edges in the human body.

This technique is based on the fact that the left hemisphere of the brain needs to send information to the right side of the body and the right hemisphere to the left side. If either of these 'communication tracts' are not adequately flowing and open then it will be impossible to access the brain's full capacity or the body's full intelligence.

The bottom line is: when our energies are crossed every system in the body and the body's healing abilities is encouraged to optimum efficiency, we are literally healthier. However, when the energies are not crossed, the healing abilities are dramatically reduced.

We are born with the energies running in a parallel pattern, homolaterally[6] down the body but when, as babies, we start to crawl; the crossover pattern and left/right brain integration really begins to take form. This is why children who do not crawl enough can develop learning difficulties. So don't just plonk your baby/grandchild in a bouncer, let it roam wild – the crawling action will enable enhanced brain function.

Back to us as adults: Nature intended that we cross crawl naturally during the course of each day: walking, running, swimming are all natural ways of consolidating that crossing pattern. However, contemporary lifestyles are increasingly sedentary. In addition, fashion footwear can prohibit good posture and, we carry heavy shoulder bags, briefcases or shopping bags which all inhibit the natural flow of the movement.

Needless to say any stress or trauma in our life can throw the pattern back into homolateral. Our body will give us hints when this happens – for example stop reading right now and see if any 'body part' is crossed – wrists, arms, ankles, legs? This is a message that the body needs/ wants to cross its energies, it yearns to run at full efficiency, it seeks balance to do so.

Body language specialists say crossed arms mean a closed off/defensive stance, but in reality, from an energetic standpoint, it can also mean that you are trying to cross the energies, albeit unconsciously, so that you can truly understand what is being said to you.

So, to summarise; doing a CROSS CRAWL can improve left and right brain integration and encourage energies to cross.

---

6 We use the word homolateral to indicate this parallel patterning. II

This in turn can:–

- Greatly improve the body's natural healing ability.

- Enhance the absorption of vitamin supplementation.

- Relieve fatigue, exhaustion and lack of motivation.

- Bring clarity to your thinking.

- Help your whole system function more efficiently.

- Improve co-ordination.

- Reduce certain learning difficulties.

- Stimulate memory.

- Pump lymphatic and cerebrospinal fluid.

- Help you feel more balanced, motivated and energised.

- Harmonise energies and increase natural self healing abilities.

- Ease depression.

- Support the immune system.

- Support and help make more effective any other treatments you may be receiving from your health-care practitioner.

It is marching on the spot
to reprogramme the body into a health supporting
crossing pattern,
without which you will never heal 100%

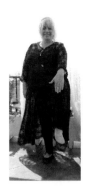
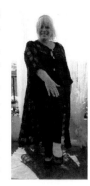

1. Lift your right arm and right leg together. Then lift your left arm and left leg together. Do you remember the Thunderbird puppets! Repeat a few times/15 seconds or so. This reflects the homolateral, parallel patterning which your brain will recognise and feel comfortable with if your energies are not crossing.

2. Now lift your right arm and left leg together [see photo on the right above] followed by left arm and right leg. i.e. diagonal/opposites together. Repeat a few times/15 seconds. This represents the cross over pattern and may feel uncomfortable until your energies reprogramme themselves into a crossing pattern.

3. Repeat

ALWAYS end on the cross over pattern

and do a few extra 'crosses' to integrate the reprogramming.

Cross Crawl every time you are waiting for the kettle to boil – let it slip effortlessly into your life and become a habit. It will be subtle, but you will definitely begin to feel the benefits within a couple of weeks.

Over the following months the body will begin to hold on to the crossover patterning as it becomes more ingrained. Any stress or trauma may send you into homolateral, but if you are cross crawling every day, you will never be in that state for more than 24 hours and therefore should not suffer from any associated symptoms.

If you have problems with mobility and cannot stand or balance to do this exercise, it can be done sitting down or even on your back in bed.

When you are striding out on a walk, make sure your body is moving in the cross/diagonal patterning and you have thumped K27 to get your energies running in the right direction – takes seconds but you will get dramatically more benefit from the exercise.

[otherwise you could be literally walking against your own flow of energy which will tire rather than refresh you.]

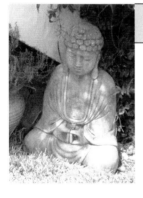

Unscrambling energy – Tibetan meditation pose

This unscrambles the energies making for clearer communication, clearer thinking, improved left/right brain integration and cheers you up in no time at all, so great for when you are feeling sad, confused or angry. It returns your energy circuits to default, reduces stress, and encourages release of past emotional baggage or trauma.

We tend to naturally sit in this position and it may be familiar to you. It is sometimes considered to be a blocking pose but in reality, if you are over-stimulated, you are naturally trying to unscramble so that you can understand more clearly, so it is the total opposite of being blocked, it is about wanting to be open and understanding.

- Sit [or stand], cross the arms over the chest with hands under the armpits, thumbs out and up. Close your eyes, breath and smile. Stay in this position until you feel calm.

- Bring your hands into prayer position and take a couple of breaths.

- Put your arms out in front of you, palms facing outwards. Feet are still crossed.

- Cross the wrists and intertwine your fingers, pull them towards you, up and under, so your clasped hands are sitting under your chin. Did you do this when you were a child? I have asked many people from different countries and most have – as children we instinctively get ourselves into positions that encourage balance.

- Close your eyes, breath and smile. Hold for as long as you want – a minute?

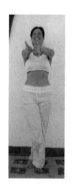 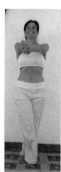 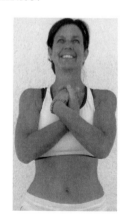

'Discombobulated'... I simply love the sound of this word although I have my doubts as to its 'official' existence, but just the sound of it manages to describe how we can all feel occasionally: Uncoordinated in both body and mind; a bit 'off'; a little 'spaced out'; stuck; not fully in the flow of life and unable to cope with the challenges life sets us.

This simple technique is a hyperlink to harmony, equilibrium and balance. It:

- connects [hooks up] two important channels of energies: Governing and Central, which in turn boosts confidence and courage

- brings clarity of thought and purpose;

- strengthens the auric field, keeping it solid and protective

- bridges the energies between the head and the body.

- enables you to feel more connected, co-ordinated, grounded and able to cope.

- stimulates Strangeflow energy

- Place the middle finger of one hand on your forehead between the eyebrows, over the 3rd Eye

- Place the middle finger of the other hand in your navel.

- With a slight pull of the skin upward on both points, close your eyes, take a deep breath and relax. [Breathe in through the nose and out through the mouth]

Stay in this position for about twenty seconds [or for however long feels right to you]

By strengthening the Governing Channel that runs up the back, you affect the spine, not only in a physical sense but also in an emotional way – literally giving you the 'backbone' to face and resolve problems and move forward in your life.

By strengthening the Central Channel that runs up the front of the torso you will be less vulnerable to absorbing other peoples' negative energies. An overdose of these can cause exhaustion and even depression.

It is a powerful tool for quickly centring yourself and has immediate neurological consequences. It has been reported to be helpful to a person starting to seizure.

Try it right now and see if you feel less discombobulated!

Integrating change with the Regulator

Tracing the Regulator Flow
takes about 30 seconds and helps the other exercises hold.
Sometimes a visual is far easier to follow – watch my clip on YouTube and see how easy this flow is.[7]

---

7 If you can't access it directly for some reason, go on my midlife goddess site, I have posted it there.

- The regulator flow is the 'co-ordinator'.

- The front (yin) and back (yang) regulator flows influence hormones, chemistry, and circulation as well as the connections among all the systems in the body. They literally turn on and co-ordinate them all.

- Relevant to any auto-immune problem [which is basically where energies are not communicating with each other or adjusting correctly].

- As it runs straight through the thyroid, it always affects it.

- Regulator helps your body adapt to endless assaults of internal and external changes.

- Hormonal imbalances and the emotional turmoil can be addressed by working with the regulator flow.

- Regulator also establishes harmonies with other people and within the environment.

- It helps you adjust to the new.

- It is essential in dealing with change.

- Being a 'strangeflow' it helps increase your 'joy in life'.

Activating the Regulator

One of the simplest ways of activating any flow is to trace it. Tracing is done with the open palms of your hands. You either touch the body/clothing or work a couple of inches over it. You can enhance the tracing by using an essential oil mix such as frankincense and lavender or holding a crystal of your choice, but these are not necessary, they are what I respectfully call 'my toy box'.

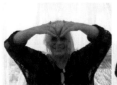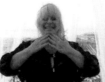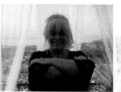

Trace the front [yin flow] on yourself

- Take a moment to stand tall, centre and earth yourself.

- Rub your hands together, place fingertips between the eyebrows.

- Trace a **HEART** around the outside of the face

- That heart sits on a **STICK** running down the front of the throat

- Cross your arms like **A GENIE** in front of you at chest level

- Uncross them, running your palms up to your shoulders so that your forearms are in a **PHARAOH** position, i.e. crossed over the chest.

- Bring hands down to the side of the breasts – a la **MARILYN** Monroe

- Smile and move hands down the front of the body – 'Oh, I'm so beautiful!'

- Move over the ribs, pelvis, thighs, knees, shins and the top of the feet, pause here

- Squeeze lateral and medial sides together [pressure on Bladder and Spleen meridians]

- End by brushing off the feet

- Come up slowly, let your abdominal muscles do the work, vertebrae by vertebrae – you may also like to swing your torso slightly in a loose figure 8.

Tracing the back flow – yang

- Palms on temples

- Do the Teddy Boy Sweep – move your palms up over the top and behind the ears and off the shoulders

- Cross your arms like a genie again, clasp the upper arm a little higher up – say an inch.

- Run your hands up the arms to the shoulders so that your forearms are again in the pharaoh position

- Then into Marilyn position on either side of your breasts

- Move hands onto the back as high as is comfortable

- Trace down the back – in at the waist and out at the hips

- Down the back of the legs and off the little toes

- Come up slowly, figure 8'ing as you come up [this helps reinforce Strangeflow energies]

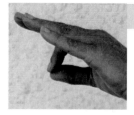

• Sit on your heels, or in lotus position or in a chair – whatever is comfortable to you.

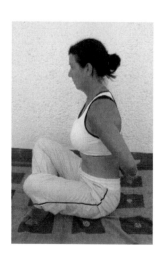

• Put your arms behind you and clasp your left wrist with your right hand and make a circle with your finger and thumb [left hand].

• Lean forward as far as you can. Stay comfortable, going a little bit further with each out breath.

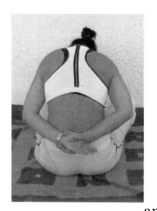

• This pose is deeply relaxing and balancing in the sense that it encourages the release of deep seated emotional baggage.

• Come out of the pose slowly and sit quietly, perhaps saying your personal prayer or read an inspirational quote and ponder upon it.

• Use this as an opportunity for a minute or two of quiet contemplation.

For example...

To those with wisdom, happiness is not about getting what you want,
it's about wanting what you've got.

A MORNING PRAYER

I give thanks and praise to the Creator who

has given me this day.

I call on the Goddess to be with me.

I ask for her peace, love and guidance.

May my guides and companions be with me, to shield, guide and protect me and may I be open to their communication.

I ask for the presence of heavenly messengers

to guide me,

and for the protection and wisdom of my ancestors.

Let the Elements and Gatekeepers of the four directions light my way. As I open to Spirit this day, show me a way to receive the abundant gifts and blessings that are bestowed upon me.

As I open to Spirit this day, show me a way to be of service to the 'greater good' of all beings

– in the most divine way.

AND SO BE IT – THANK YOU

This was given to me by a friend many many years ago.
If anyone knows who actually wrote it, please let me know.

Side bend with St36

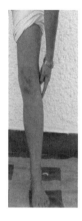

This bend opens up the whole area around your middle [belt area] and creates space for energy to flow through all the organs in the mid torso and up the gallbladder and spleen meridians. Holding Stomach 36 points gives you a burst of energy. This acupoint is called the 3 Mile points and is one of acupunctures 'master points' – Go to the knee, place your opposite palm around the leg with your index finger along the bottom edge of the kneecap the point will be under the 3rd or 4th finger - flex and point the foot to find the point in the muscle belly 2 fingers to the outside [lateral] of the centre of the shinbone... it will probably be tender

This is a very powerful and frequently used acupuncture point [I think of it as one point does all] that is particularly helpful for a number of imbalances in the abdominal region as well as strengthening the blood and the energy in the stomach meridian.

It is great for stable grounding in a mad world. Work these points when you feel tired yet need to carry to, it will revive you – but don't abuse it!

There is a legend that says a general in an ancient Chinese army needed his troops to march more, but they were all exhausted from fighting and marching for so many weeks, they stopped and refused to go further. The general ordered his army doctor to stimulate St36 on every soldier – legend has it that the troops marched for another 3 miles and reached their destination –

hence the point is called *Three Mile Point.*

Working with Stomach meridian is about self care, trusting in the mystery of life and letting go of unnecessary anxiety – relax and enjoy the ride, stop worrying – you can't change the past and who knows what tomorrow will bring – live fully grounded in the moment.

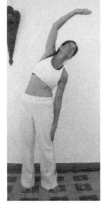

•   Stand with feet firmly on the ground, about hip width apart

•   Bend your knees slightly and imagine yourself rooting down into the earth, feeling grounded and stable

•   Close your eyes and place your palms on your thighs and take a couple of deep breaths and smile. Come into the present moment.

•   Straighten up and bring your hands into prayer position in front of your chest, put a little pressure against your Thymus while you there – just 10 seconds.

•   Take your right hand onto your right leg on the St 36 points, apply a little pressure.

•   At the same time take your left arm up over your head and bend sideways. Make sure you are not tipping forward or backwards. Success is not how far over you go, it is feeling a good, painless stretch down the whole of your left side. [if you prefer, you can do this technique sitting in a chair].

•   Stay in that position for 30 seconds

•   Come back to centre and prayer position – press against the Thymus

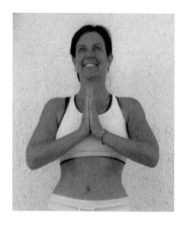

• Repeat on the other side, again hold the pose for 30 seconds

• Come back to centre and prayer position – press against the Thymus

• Don't forget, stay smiling throughout.

The PC stretch

This stretch opens up the front of the body creating space for blood, lymph, energy to flood the organs in the front torso. It squeezes the kidneys, which are then refreshed when you straighten. Invigorates these organs and enhances their efficiency.

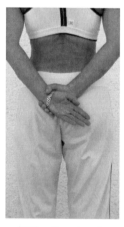

You will also be creating space for all the front flowing meridians, penetrating flow and the chakras... suffice to say, with one single stretch you are working out a lot of energy systems and their accompanying organs! The beginning stretch opens the lungs which are often associated with trusting and letting go.

Enjoy this stretch, especially if you have been sitting at a computer all day – it is an effective all rounder and don't forget, smile while you do it.

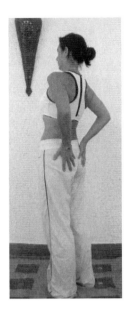

With all respect, Prince Charles is famous for standing with his arms behind his back – so start in that position with the right hand clasping the left hand and the left hand forming a 'O' with the forefinger and thumb. Pull back and down a bit until you feel a stretch across your chest and front of shoulders. [you will remember this from Yoga Mudra].

Hold in that position for 30 seconds [it takes that long for the brain to instruct the muscles to let go] – keep your eyes closed and tune in to what is happening in that chest area.

Place the palms of your hands over the top of your bottom with the heels over the sacrum area, fingers pointing down the legs. Now arch your back and bend backwards as far as is comfortable, hold for as long as is comfortable.

Straighten up slowly, wrap your right hand over your spleen, located under your left breast, and left hand around your upper arm and give yourself a little hug [you are connecting Spleen and Triple Warmer which has the effect of reducing stress and increasing your ability to deal with problems and enhance your immunity].

Obviously if you have any lower back problem, leave this portion of the exercise out, or ask your healthcare provider if it is suitable for you.

Never, ever go into pain, you defeat the whole object of an exercise and may do yourself harm.

In some healing cultures the spine is considered the centre of your health universe, if it is flexible and the energy free flowing that will reflect throughout the entire body. Governing [courage to move forward in life, your backbone] and Bladder [letting go of unnecessary fear] meridians sit neatly along it and are directly affected. It makes sense therefore to gently stretch and create space for energy to flow up and down this crucial column. If healthy, every aspect of your well being will be positively affected.

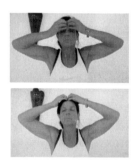

PART 1

Open up the area: start with fingertips on your forehead and pull apart, working up over an imaginary central line over the top and down the back of the head and neck, then down the spine to the sacrum and then brush off down both legs.

Come up slowly *imagining* horizontal figure 8's over the back of your legs, bottom and back.

PART 2

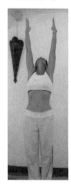

Reach up with your arms above your head and gently bend forward as far as is comfortable. Hold for 30 seconds. Come up slowly, vertebrae by vertebrae, using your abdominal girdle to do so. It does not matter how far forward you bend, it is feeling a stretch along the entire back, hamstrings and possibly calves.

PART 3

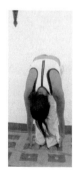

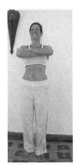
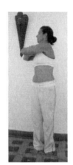

Spinal twist. Clasp your forearms in front of you like a genie at chest level.

Keeping your hips facing forwards, inhale and as you exhale slowly swing your body around to the right as far as is comfortable, hold for 10 seconds, come back to the centre and repeat on the other side.

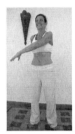

Come back to standing tall with knees gently bent, arms down by your side, swing slowly round to each side and as momentum grows your arms will wrap around your body.

Slow down and come back to centre and tune into your spine – can you feel the energy running through it now?

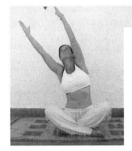

Sitting spinal workout

Has the same benefits as the spinal workout

• Sit comfortably on the floor in any variation of the lotus position, back straight. Reach arms up above your head and bend sideways towards the point where the ceiling joins the wall. Repeat on the other side.

• Return to centre

• Lean forward, arms out on the floor in front of

35

you, walk the hands to the left, come back to centre and walk them to the right. Come back to centre and straighten up.

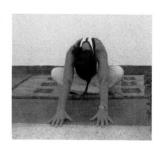

- Bring chin to chest and stay in that position for 30 seconds.

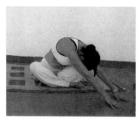

• Sit up straight

• Bring your feet so that the soles face each other, knees pointing to the side.

• Grasp feet and bend forward from the hips, keeping the back straight.

Imagine you are taking your chest to the floor, not your head. You may only move two or three inches, that is fine, the stretch you achieve and the benefit to your body is every bit as effective as if you had your head on the floor!

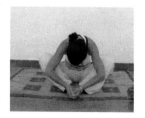

- Stay in this forward bend for 30 seconds and come up slowly. I always remember being told, in Trager that the longer one stays in a stretch the more effective it will be as it takes the brain about 20-30 seconds to feel 'safe' to instruct a muscle to 'let go'. Muscles can do nothing without an instruction from the brain, so we need to 'talk' to the brain to achieve a real stretch, this is why paying attention and focussing on what a stretch is doing to your body makes it more effective.

- Sit quietly and massage firmly along the inside of each foot [in reflexology this reflects your entire spine] note and linger on any points that are tender.

[If you are not a reflexologist – Google British School of Reflexology and download their foot map, then you know exactly what you are massaging].

Atlas shrugged

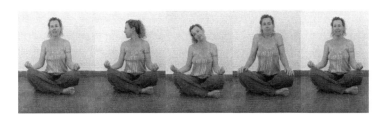

A variation on the classic neck roll that creates space in the neck area for energy to flow, thereby affecting the arms, hands, shoulder area and of course the head.

Best to do this sitting down the first few times as it can make you feel a little dizzy as you clear muscle tightness and energy congestion in the area, allowing an increase in blood flow.

Start by massaging along the base of the skull – best to use your thumbs, which mean your fingers are over the back of your head – linger on any areas that seem to be tender or tight – these can often cause tension headaches. The Body Shop used to make little plastic pads that fitted over your thumbs and were great for massaging this area. Take your time on this part of the technique, it can release a lot of tension and feel invigorating as blood begins to circulate in the area.

Move down to the neck and place your fingertips on either side of the spine and pull apart, paying particular attention to the area where a necklace sits. Again this creates space not only for energy to move but cerebral spinal fluid and blood, thereby bathing the brain in oxygen and nutrients.

Sit with hands in front of you in your lap and bring your chin to your chest and stay in that position until you can feel the stretch down either side of your spine reaching your sacral area – if you need an extra hand, place your forearms on the back of your head, don't push down, just let the weight stretch out the muscles.

Bring your head up slowly look round to the right and hold for 20 seconds.

Come back to the centre and then look round to the left and hold for 20 seconds.

Back to centre and bring your right ear down to the right shoulder [NOT your shoulder up to your ear].

Back to centre and bring your left ear down to the left shoulder.

End with a huge shrug and release.

You will note I make no mention of throwing the head backwards, this is because compressing the vertebrae in this way can be dangerous to do especially if you have any weakness whatsoever in that area.

One of the fundamental beliefs of energy medicine is that wherever there is pain in the body, there will also be 'stagnation' of some kind: blood, lymph, energy, nerve connections – nothing will be flowing or operating smoothly. Energy especially becomes 'stuck' and can even begin to move backwards along the meridians, causing toxic build up. This, combined with years of wear and tear and probable abuse, results in stiffness and pain, especially in the joints, back, neck and shoulders.

Hairbrush tapping is the equivalent to 50 little fingers are stimulating the area:–

1. Buy a hairbrush, the style with hard plastic 'spikes'

2. With a light wrist, gently tap all over the joint area with the spiky side of the hairbrush.

3. Tapping can be in any direction, speed or pattern you wish.

4. The area should be covered with material – ideally do not tap directly onto skin, it can be a little ir-ritating for sensitive skins.

5. Tap for 10 seconds or 10 minutes – whatever feels good or is convenient.

6. Rub, in an anticlockwise circle, over the painful area with either the heel of the hand or with the fingers. An anticlockwise direction tends to 'lift' pain out of an area. You may like to use some oil to help the process – a few drops of the essential oils Black Pepper and Sweet Marjoram diluted in a carrier such as Sweet Almond Oil, smell divine as they warm and relax the area. Creams that contain Wintergreen, menthol, eucalyptus, camphor etc.,

are useful tools in your arsenal against rigidity and pain.

7. To finish, 'brush off' the limb with the flat palms of your hands. For example, if you were tapping the knee joint you would end by placing both palms on either side of the knee and with a light pressure, slide the hands down to the feet and come off the toes.

8. End by tracing Figure 8's [Tibetan healing symbol] over the area.

It is inexpensive and takes very little time or effort. Many of my clients over the years have used this deceptively simple technique and have experienced fantastic results: return of sensation in an area, reduced pain, increased movement etc., My teacher and friend Donna Eden tapped away her MS [sounds remarkable? Google her or read her book Energy Medicine for the full story]

Keep the brush in eyesight, maybe by the bed, television, and computer – wherever you will *see* it. That way it will remind you to tap. If it is stuck away in a drawer, believe me, you will forget to do it!

Spinal flush

We are all familiar with the body's lymphatic system, garbage disposal at its best, key to our immunity, helping counter conditions ranging from colds to cancer. The lymphatic system is bigger than the circulatory system, but does not have a heart to pump the lymph around the body; it relies on gravity and exercise/

movement. With our increasingly sedentary lifestyles, the system can become sluggish and less effective in clearing toxins from certain parts of the body. When this happens the 'garbage' can accumulate and cause very real problems.

To maintain a healthy lymphatic system: move, walk, body brush, drink water, get a massage and a daily 'Spinal Flush'.

"What is a Spinal Flush?" I hear you ask. It is simply a firm massage along either side of the spine. Through clothes or directly on skin, it stimulates certain 'neurolymphatic reflex points' that trigger the garbage disposal system into activity and encourage the efficient removal of toxins from the body and strengthen immunity. You will feel more energized and optimistic as the body begins to rid itself of stagnant energies and emotional residue. It also stimulates the cerebrospinal fluid, clearing your head. If you feel the very first signs of a cold coming on, a Spinal Flush can stimulate your immunity enough to nip it in the bud. In fact, if you did this every day to each other, you may not even catch a cold in the first place!

It is a great technique for partners as it quickly dissolves built up stress and takes the edge off any 'emotional overreaction' [an understated way of saying things getting a little heated and you are about to either become a foulmouthed fishwife, go into a tight lipped sulk or walk out the door!]. So, rather than head towards an argument and divorce proceedings, give each other a spinal flush, an inexpensive form of marriage counselling without words!

If any of the points feel sore, unless there is an obvious reason, such as a bruise, injury or medical condition, the soreness indicates that the point, and its corresponding organ, need a bit of attention, so linger on the point a little longer. However, if you are recovering from an illness or suffer an autoimmune problem, you may find a lot of the points are sore. If this is the case, go easy so as not to overwhelm the system.

To do the Spinal Flush takes about a minute, but is so enjoyable you may well be pleading 'don't stop!'.

Lie face down, or stand 3-4 feet from a wall and lean into it with your hands supporting you at chest level. This positions your body to remain stable while your partner applies pressure to your back.

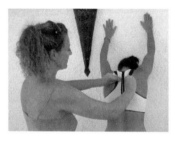

Your partner massages the points down either side of your spine, using the thumbs, fingers or knuckles and applying body weight to get strong pressure but no rough, jerky or sudden movements. Massage from the bottom of the neck all the way down to the bottom of the sacrum. Go down the notches between the vertebrae and deeply massage each point for a few seconds, moving the skin in a circular motion with strong pressure but ensuring that the pressure is comfortable. This technique should not feel painful. Make sure neither of you are holding your breath.

Upon reaching your sacrum, your partner can repeat the massage or complete it by 'sweeping' the energies down your body, from your shoulders, and with an open hand, all the way down your legs and off your feet, 2-3 times.

Each of these points relate to a specific energy meridian/organ but do not be concerned about missing one, just work between all the notches and give a little extra time to any that feel 'sore'.

If you dwell a bit on the points just above the sacrum, they relate to Bladder which governs 'fear' which is an emotion that often stops us stepping out with courage and doing what our heart wants to do.

I suppose I should say, please use your common sense and do not do a Spinal Flush if there is even a whisper of spinal injury, bruising or problems in the area. If in any doubt check with your healthcare practitioner.

Okay, so what happens if you do not have a willing partner? Then, two tennis balls in a sock are going to be your best friends!

Place two tennis balls in a sock and tie the end tightly. Lie on your back with knees bent and feet flat on the floor. Raise your body up slightly and place the balls under the top of the spine. The spine itself will sit comfortably between each ball. Pressure should never be applied directly to the bone itself, but to the muscles on either side of the spine. Lower your weight on to the ball and wriggle around so it massages the neurolymphatic reflex points.

Alternatively, you can just lie on top of the balls and after about 30 seconds you will begin to feel the back relax and the points 'opening'. Do this down the entire length of the spine, spending a little extra time on any sore spots.

If getting up and down from the floor is not easy for you, an excellent variation [in fact it is my favourite] is to place the balls on a wall, ideally on a corner, or door jam. Feet should be placed about 18" away from the wall [the further away the more pressure is applied to the back]. Lean your full body weight against the balls. Bend knees to manoeuvre them up and down the spine, wriggle around and pay attention to the sore points.

Sit against the balls on a plane, it helps reduce back pain, you might get a few funny looks but your back will benefit.

There is another technique with these tennis balls that you might like to try: place them under the head so the weight of the head rests on the balls. Ideally positioned in a small indentation your will find half way up the skull, on the centre line. If you don't have the tennis balls you can rest your head on your two clasped fists, but make sure it is not causing tension in your muscles. This reduces stress and fear in the body. If it feels a bit too strong for you, just use the palm of your hand.

Zip up and sew up

The line up the front of our torso is the Central pathway of energy and could be considered rather like a sponge that soaks up all the energies we come up against; people and environmental. It is how we interact. Fantastic if all that energy is brimming with positivity but what happens if you are coming up against energies of depression, fear, anger, anxiety, stress? Well the bad news is, if your Central pathway is not strong, you will just suck up all that energy and often retain it in your torso where it can get up to all sorts of energetic mischief.

The good news is that it takes seconds to empty it out and strengthen it so that you can walk the earth without being 'soaked' in negativity. It is also great for expelling any pent up anger, irritability or general huffiness!

Stand tall, close your eyes and take some deep breaths, really expanding the ribcage. This in itself begins the balancing process.

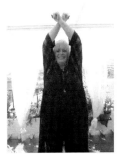
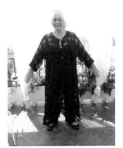

Massage firmly the area beneath your right breast, exactly where the under-wire of a bra sits. Do this for 15 seconds, it will be tender but keep the pressure firm. This is a neurolymphatic reflex point that helps balance the Liver. Now for the Gallbladder: let both arms hang down the side of the body in a relaxed way, directly under where the middle fingers hang are the points that you need to massage firmly to begin to balance Gallbladder.

Place hands over your head, arms straight, fists clenched, wrists crossed.

Breathing out, bring hands down quickly and with force, uncrossing and taking them out to the side of the thighs with fingers now outstretched, not clenched.

While doing this, imagine a line that runs down the centre of the body, from mouth to the genital area. Imagine this line opening up, becoming 'unzipped' and any anger, rage, irritation, or negative energetic 'gunk' that has been lurking inside finally spilling out into the earth.

At the same time breathe out with a hissing sound and imagine all those toxic emotions, energies and thoughts spilling out on your breath.

Repeat 3 times

You are now 'open' and it is important to zip up that Central Meridian so that toxic energies that may be around you can no longer enter and cause disruption. This zip up boosts confidence and positivity and clears your thoughts.

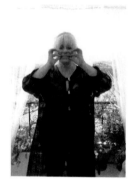

Simply place your hand at the bottom of the meridian [between your legs]. Take a deep in-breath and simultaneously move your hand up the centre of the body to your lower lip and 'lock it' by lightly tweaking the sides of your mouth.

As you do this, think of calmness, forgiveness and tranquillity being zipped up inside.

Do this 3 times and end by 'sewing up' i.e. tracing a horizontal Figure of 8 up the centre line, rather like an old fashioned Victorian corset.

This will give you a wonderful protection against external energies entering your body; against some of the stresses of life triggering unnecessary anger. It does not stifle you; you can still give out care, warmth, attention and love.

Hold top and bottom of spine + imagine 8's

Put your left hand around the back of your neck, gently cupped.

Put your right hand [or fingertips] over your sacral area – wherever is comfortable.

Close your eyes and hold this position, imaging horizontal Figure 8's running up and down the spine between your hands.

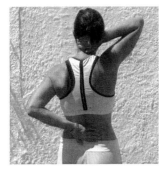

This helps activate the flow of blood, energy and cerebral spinal fluid along the spine to the brain and also activate Strangeflow energy in the body which helps you deal with change and begins to bring a sense of joy back into your life, more specifically with this exercise you will be stimulating Bridge Flow energy, this simply means that you will be enhancing all areas of 'communication' in your life, it literally bridges systems, people, worlds, emotions, healings – anything and everything.

- It connects the sides of the body

- It connects the front and back [yin and yang] of the body

- It enhances polarities

- It heightens intuition

- It improves communications with others

- It always works for the 'highest good'

- It enables 'stuck' energy to move

Top Tip

Gently holding these two simple points on the side of your head until you feel a pulse under your fingertips improves your immunity and helps you process and

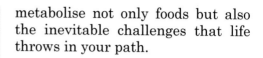

metabolise not only foods but also the inevitable challenges that life throws in your path.

Deeply relaxing in only 30 seconds.

They are powerful neurovascular points and holding them draws the blood to them [hence the pulse] activating the organ [in this case Spleen] associated with them.

Positioned on the side of the skull, 2 fingers above the top tip of your ear.

Cleopatra

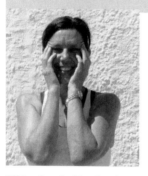

I think we all do this, look at this photo of me, which was unintentional but I obviously needed it!

Rest your chin on the heels of your hands with the fingertips placed in a line running from edge of eye to ear – rather like Elizabeth Taylor's make up in Cleopatra.

Sit there for 30 seconds, smile and count your blessings – literally feel an attitude of gratitude.

What's happening? You are balancing the neurovascular points associated with Stomach [on the jaw line] and on the Cleopatra line: Governing, Triple Warmer and Kidney.

What does that do? It reduces stress, anxiety and fear and increases courage and your ability to process problems.

If you are a therapist, do this hold, hands will be reversed. Simply hold for a few minutes and your client will be snoring.

Tummy tucking

How long is it since you could look down and see your pubic hair? If you are in possession of a bellowing Buddha belly, this for you. I will not bore you with all the scientific blurb but it is a fact that as we get older our hormonal dance and metabolism slows down and seemingly overnight fat sneaks up and ambushes our waist, abdominal muscles seem to disappear resulting in an endearing little Buddha Belly, or as my cats think of it: a comfy cushion to paw and curl up on when it gets chilly. There are few exceptions, even skinny minnies and gym junkies can fall foul to thick waist syndrome.

Beware, buried deep underneath that cute BB could be a little too much visceral fat which may cause serious health problems [*TIP: if the flab does not drift down to the sides when you lie down, it it stays solid on top [like a beer belly], it could be a sign that it is Cortisol related fat – this can only be reduced by exercise*]. The midsection matters – as a rule of thumb, if your waist measures more than 35inches you may have a problem and should consider a regular exercise routine and healthy diet to reduce the fat in this area.

Based on Pilates, this is one of the simplest techniques to do and can, if done daily, be one of the most effective [physically]. It will strengthen the abdominal girdle, which in turn gives you a slimmer appearance. In addition, strengthening these muscles relieves stress on the lower back, improves overall posture and creates space for key organs to function and energies to flow. It encourages the flow of cerebral spinal fluid and energy in the Governing vessel, providing 'backbone' to move forward in life.

Remember those days when we used to try and get into skinny tight jeans and had to pull our stomachs in tightly to do up the zip, often with the aid of a metal coat hanger? Well, Tummy tucking is very similar...

- Pull up the muscles of the pelvic floor and draw back your navel back towards the spine, as far as you can. It is like pulling up your internal zip rather than the jeans.

- Now release it 50% and hold that taut feeling. This is how your abdominals should be all the time.

- Keep breathing and doing whatever you are doing.

No doubt, within seconds, you will lose the 'tuck' – don't worry, just keep doing it all day, every day and it will slowly begin to re-educate and tone the muscles. One very useful tactic is to stick little yellow 'post it notes' all around your home, office and car. The rule is:- every time you see a yellow sticker you 'tummy tuck'! Don't worry if it seems difficult at first, I couldn't even find a muscle to pull in when I started, but now I can TT with the best of them!

The Buddha belly swish

Works on an 'energetic' level clearing stagnant energy away from the belt area, this in turn will have a positive impact on the body's physical ability to let go of midsection fat and stimulate organs in that area. You will also be working over part of the Penetrating and Belt flows which are associated with joy, so smile and feel good while you do this.

- Place palms of hands on both kidneys and bring round to the front of the body and off with a clap.

- Breathe out as you do this and imagine all the fat coming out of your body on that long exhalation and being squeezed out of waist area by the hands.

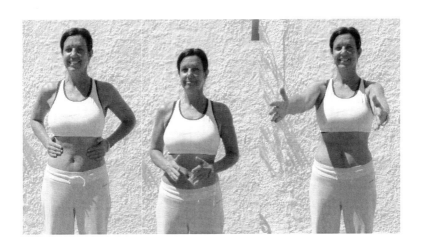

The Inverted 'V'

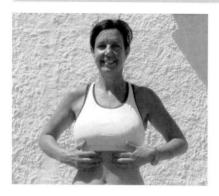

Anything that reduces stress and tension and allows energy to move through the midsection will help clear toxins from the area and stimulate metabolism: Stretching is excellent. There is also a key pressure point located in the Solar Plexus area, right in the centre of the inverted 'V' formed by the front of the ribcage. Press your fingers in and up firmly on this area, lean back a bit to expose the ribs and massage strongly for 10 seconds along the edge of the ribcage, it may be tender but it will begin to release stagnant energy and encourage a flat stomach. Do before and after any abdominal exercises to maximise benefits.

Ear Ear!

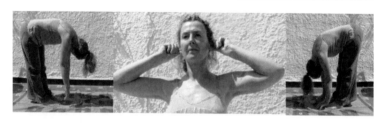

I shouldn't really say this but I can't resist – here is a great party trick.:

Gently lean forward to touch your toes, go as far as you can and note where you land.

Using your fingers and thumbs vigorously rub the entire ear lobe [on both ears] until they are hot and red, really give them a good massage.

Now do that forward bend again – hey presto, look how much more flexible you are.

Why?

The ear is said to be a reflection of your entire body, imagine a little foetus curled up in there. There is a discipline called auricular acupuncture that works the body through points on the ear and by massaging over all these points you are giving your entire body a workout, including the muscles and ligaments, hence your ability to stretch more after an ear rub.

They are also your antennae to the world and receivers of information so, if you are at workshop, meeting or wherever you need to keep 'an ear open' do a quick rub to move the energy and you will be surprised how much easier it is to take in and assimilate that information as it improves listening, concentration and comprehension.

Eye Eye!

One of the simplest exercises for the eyes is tracing a horizontal Figure 8. We sometimes do this instinctively when we doodle 8's in whatever direction.

· Encourages the movement of energy behind the eyes

· Encourages right and left brain integration

· Improves co ordination

1. Sit in a relaxed position and look straight ahead.

2. Trace a horizontal Figure of 8 with eyes, really reaching up into the corners.

You may find it easier to follow the path of your fingers...

1. Form a triad with the thumb and first two fingers of one hand.

2. Hold that triad about 12 inches away from the bridge of your nose.

3. Trace the Figure of 8 and let your eyes follow, whilst keeping the head facing straight ahead, centred and relaxed.

Illeocecal valve stretch in the shower

It resets the Illeocecal Valve, which, located on the right hand side of the tum, is a one way valve that allows digested food to pass from the small to the large intestine for further processing. It stops waste materials from backing up into the small intestine [rather like a backed up sink drain] Simple, but when it goes wrong it can cause huge problems of toxicity in the body. What can cause it to go wrong? Dehydration, bad eating behaviours such as under chewing food, eating too quickly, eating the wrong foods: sodas, alcohol, caffeine, sugar etc., and of course, emotional stress of any kind.

Whether the valve is stuck open or closed you can use the same correction technique. Problems such as eczema, bronchitis, digestive disorders, lower backaches can all clear up after this valve's functioning is restored. Best done in the shower with soapy hands, resetting this valve can reap huge benefits and takes less than 30 seconds!

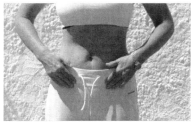

1. *Place the right hand on the right hip bone with the little finger at it's inside edge. Your hand is now over the valve.*

2. *Place the left hand at the corresponding spot on the inside edge of the left hipbone. This is the houston valve, resetting both valves creates a symmetry between them.*

3. *Firmly massage in a circular motion and then slowly drag the fingers of each hand up six to seven inches with a deep inhalation. Keep the pressure of the drag as deep as you can.*

4. *Shake the energy off your fingers with the out breath and return to the original position. Repeat about 4 times*

5. *End by dragging your fingers downward one time with pressure*

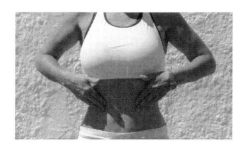

Creating space in the back of the legs

Sit on the floor with your legs out in front of you, feet flexed [or stand and do it]. Massage the back of the legs, along the centre line and pull out from that centre line to the edges, opening up the back of the leg, creating space for energy to flow freely through the large hamstring and calf muscles which when tight can contribute to backache.

You will also be stimulating the flow of Bladder energy which in the Traditional Chinese philosophy sits in Water Element which governs new beginnings, creativity and fear. So, on both a physical and emotional level you will walk forward with ease.

Open the Gaits

The gaits – the channels between the tendons on the top of the feet – are often forgotten in our healthcare regimes. They can become stiff and inflexible through mechanical stresses: injury, bad fitting shoes, walking on cobbles or uneven surfaces. This can cause a disturbance in the normal co ordination of the muscles used in walking and over time can result in knee, hip or back pain and general over tiredness. In reflexology this area of the foot relates to the breasts and ribs. In energy medicine that whole area is associated with numerous meridians: kidney on the ball of the foot [as above so below]; spleen, liver, gallbladder, stomach and bladder. So working the gaits can affect almost the entire body.

Feet should hold a certain polarity to allow us to absorb energy from the surface of the earth, this can often get reversed through flying, excessive driving or anything that separates our feet from the ground; thus denying our bodies an essential source of energy nourishment.

So, however you view them, the feet deserve a little loving attention from time to time.

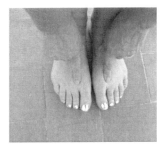

A simple massage can work wonders: Pinch each gait softly two or three times before vigorously working the area: stretch the feet from heel to ball, flex and point each foot, massage outwards, inwards, diagonally and then firmly up between each tendon: start from the gap between the big and second toe and deeply press/massage along the channel up over the top of the foot to the bottom of the leg, repeat along the other 3 channels. Rub the bottom and side of each foot too. If you have a stainless steel spoon handy, rub the smooth edge up the sole of your feet from heel to toe two or three times. If you are by the sea, end with walking along the shoreline, feet in water, relishing each step. If you have a garden, sit with your feet on the earth for a few minutes.

The gaits are also involved in our personal 'electrical' system and essential to our sense of emotional stability: if they are congested or out of balance in any way, then just the simple act of walking can not only adversely affect the muscles of the body but also our sense of being centred, being earthed.

Anything to do with the feet can also be associated with our personal perception of the future: after all, our feet carry us forward in life. If, either consciously or unconsciously, we fear that future, for example: loss, loneliness, poverty etc., it can reflect in the health of our feet.

So, once a day open the gaits wide! Use a warm, earthy oil to massage the entire foot area, I love the nuttiness of organic Argan oil or a pure local olive oil – add a few drops of your favourite essential oil to enhance the treatment [it will be absorbed rapidly into the body via the soles of the feet]. Rub the spoon from heel to toe. End by sitting on your heels [or cushion on your heels] to stretch out the front of the feet and if you really want to go the whole hog twirl a multi faceted glass crystal or polo mint magnet over the end of each toe to stimulate the flow of energy along those energy pathways then calm by gently stroking each foot from ankle to toenails and off.

Barefoot

Was the invention of the shoe a good or bad thing? Some say it was the start of us becoming less connected with mother Earth and the source of energy she provides. As we ride in cars, fly in planes, live in high rises are we becoming 'unearthed'?

A simple remedy is to connect to the Earth once a day for 10 minutes – walk barefoot on the grass, sand, earth – try and find a patch of the planet that you can set your feet upon and imagine roots burrowing down into the earth though which you absorb energy into all your systems.

Pilot Light

Our Chakra system is a prime example of teamwork, each spinning wheel of energy working with the others.

We tend to dwell on the main 7 Chakras, but there are many more and four of the most important ones are located in each knee and ankle and in my mind act like a pilot light for the entire system.

If these are spinning, open and healthy then energy can run up the legs, from the earth and feed the main chakras.

Our chakra system influences every part of our body with the key focus on our emotions and endocrine systems. If these four mini chakras are stagnant, blocked, congested – whatever word you wish to use to signify they are not open and fully working – then your entire chakra energy system will be sluggish and this in turn will reflect predominantly on your emotional well being.

A simple daily routine will keep your chakra 'pilot light' flickering:

- Sit comfortably in a chair and alternately flex and point your feet – remember ballet classes? Then rotate your feet [together] in a clockwise direction and then in an anticlockwise direction – spend about 20/30 seconds doing this.

- Hairbrush tap [spikes of a plastic hairbrush] all around each of the joints.

- Brush off from mid thigh to feet

- End by figure 8'ing each joint.

I love this one, and kids do it automatically.

It opens the hip and pelvic area and can release the lower back area.

It sets up a pumping action that enhances cerebro-spinal fluid circulation increasing alertness, clarity and left and right brain integration, reinforcing the cross over patterning of energy necessary for healing.

It releases tension along the spine and influences the flow of Central and Bladder meridians so helps us let go of fear and have backbone in facing life.

It can be done on the floor or bed, when reading or watching television – the windscreen wiper motion feels great, it is 'playful' and lifts the mood.

Please use your common sense and if you suffer lower back or knee pain, consult your healthcare professional before you do this technique.

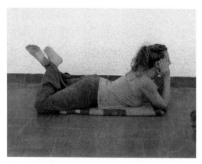

- Lie face down with your head turned to one side and resting on your hands. Or, if you are reading or watching TV your chin will be resting on the heels of your hands.

- Bend your knees so that the lower legs is at right angles with the floor.

- Now swing the feet outward and inward at whatever speed you feel is comfortable.

- Alternate which foot crosses in front

- Get your own rhythm going and keep scissor kicking for as long as you like – say a minimum of 2 minutes.

- When you are finished, roll over onto your back and tune into your body and sense how it feels.

Lung and Large Intestine reflex points

Massage firmly the breastbone from top to bottom – you are working special lymphatic reflex points to the lung area. So great if you are a smoker, have a cough or suffer from any disease in the lungs. You only need to do it for 10 seconds or so, but make sure you do it firmly.

The Large Intestine points are on the outside of your thigh, exactly where the seams of your trousers sit. Dig in firmly. It can help any problem with the Large Intestine, such as constipation [make sure you go from hip to knee direction] loose bowels [go from knee to hip].

In Traditional Chinese Medicine, these two meridians sit in Metal Element, associated with grief and letting go. None of us can escape the grip of grief in our lives and we all need to let go of some emotional baggage before we can truly move forward.

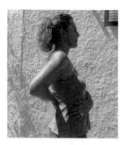 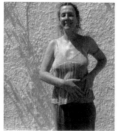 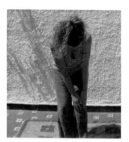

This little exercise opens up and stimulates the flow of energy around the waist. It works on many levels. It

- Connects the energies of the top part of the body and the bottom part – we need that connection and balance, not only in a physical sense but also in an energetic sense – handling the balance between being 'cosmically connected' [inspired, some may call it 'off with the fairies'] and firmly grounded [paying the mortgage on time]. We have to exist in the real world.

- It keeps the chakras and meridians flowing, which reflects on every single system of the body. Particularly the second and third chakras which is related to our sense of responsibility.

- It can be associated with the illeocecal valve, digestive problems in general, lower back pain and varicose veins.

With fingers spread, circle the hands around the left side of the body at the waist. Pull from the back of the body to the front, all the way across the belly and to the other side. Pull not only at the waist, but above and below it as well.

Do this several times with some pressure. Then firmly slide both hands down the right leg and off the foot. Repeat on the other side of the body.

Eastern Master points that do it all

These take a little time to learn but are well worth the effort – go on You Tube and you can see me demonstrating them, sometimes a visual is easier to understand than a diagram.

If you accept the premise that when things go wrong with your body, it can always be traced back to STRESS either causing or exacerbating the problem: then doesn't it make sense to find something that reduces that stress response?

So, what if I told you that there was a little sequence of acupuncture holding points that, if you do every day, for a minimum of 4 minutes, will reduce the harmful impact that stress has on your body. They can help *anything*: which means you never need feel 'helpless' again with these big bold points to fall back on!

If it was a tablet, I would be a very rich lady right now. It is not, but it IS something you can do for yourself, and this is how:

- Locate the points described below, don't worry too much about pin-point accuracy, if you go to the approximate location your fingertips will cover the actual point.

- Use fingers rather than thumbs.

- Hold the points lightly

- Hold them until you feel a strong pulse under your fingertips [this is a sign that blood is moving into the point] this can take 20 seconds or 20 minutes depending upon how chronic the problem is.

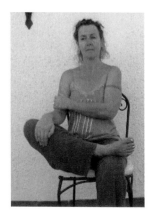

OK so let's get down to the nitty-gritty – here are the points to hold, for those of you who work with energy you will recognise them as the Triple Warmer sedation points, but you know, it doesn't matter what they are called, it is what they do, that is so important!

Hold Triple Warmer 10 above the back centre of the elbow together with Stomach 36, three finger widths below the kneecap for about a minute on each side of the body, or until you feel the pulse.

Hold the control points, Triple Warmer 2 on the back of the hand in the web between the 4th and 5th finger, and Bladder 66 on the outside of the foot at the base of the toe, for about 1.5 – 2 minutes on each side of the body.

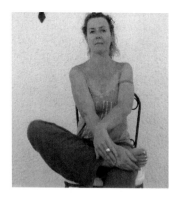

While you do this, smile to yourself and tune into your body as you feel the energy change.

Eskimo kiss

You can do this with your partner, or use your finger: rub the end of your nose from side to side. This simple little technique stimulates the flow of energy around your body. Smile while you do it.

Meridian shake up

Stand tall, with arms loosely by your side and knees relaxed [i.e. not locked]. Smile and start jumping up and down but keep your feet on the ground, think of yourself as a rag doll being shaken up: you are shaking yourself and in doing so shaking up the energy in every single pathway in the body. This means you are invigorating the entire body.

Do for one minute then stand quietly and feel the tingle of the energy moving.

Alternate arm push

One of my favourite exercises is Donna Eden's 'Connecting Heaven and Earth' take a look on www.youtube.com/watch?v=U6Yg_yRvmrg this is a great clip of Donna doing this exercise when she came to visit me in Spain.

Another version of this is worth trying as well, to ring the changes so to speak.

It helps the crossing pattern in the body, necessary for good healing.

It stretches the torso and stimulates flow of energy to all the organs.

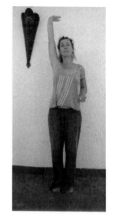

It stretches the Spleen meridian and enhances immunity

- Stand with feet together and your hands clenched loosely into fists at waist level with the palms facing upwards.

- Open the right fist and lift the arm up to the heavens with the palm facing up, look up at that hand.

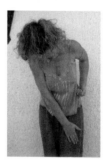

- Turn the torso to the left, keeping the arm up

- Drop the right palm and bend forward touching the outside of the left leg [wherever is comfortable] with the right palm

- Centre yourself in the forward bend and come up slowly, using your abdominal girdle to lift you, and letting your arm come up the outside of your right thigh.

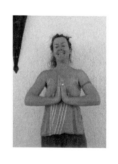

- Repeat using the left arm in the opposite direction.

- Do two or three times and end with your hands in prayer position against your chest, pressing slightly into the Thymus for 10 seconds.

- Release and bring your hands up in front of your face [still in prayer position] and up over your head then opening into a wide arc bringing them down to your sides. [This action can help bring down blood pressure].

- Smile.

Finger push-ups and pull offs

This stimulates energy related to your lung, large intestine, pericardium, triple warmer, heart and small intestine – so it gets a lot!

Place palms together, then keeping them together press the fingertips together and lower them. Very difficult to do at first as you are moving in a way that is not 'everyday'.

Great for stiff fingers – put a post it note on your computer and when you are not typing do it a few times a day to keep energies flowing through your digits.

End by pulling energy along each finger and off the end. Feels great after a long day at the keyboard. At college we used to pull the energy off between the gap created between index and middle finger and make a 'popping' sound as we came of the finger being pulled. It makes you smile, try it.

Heaven rushing in

Stand facing the sun or the moon, open your arms, take a moment to ground yourself, place your hands on your thighs, knees gently bent and feel roots running down

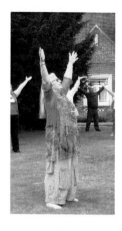

from the soles of your feet into the earth.

Arch your back opening your chest to the skies really stretching arms backwards and downwards [we tend to do this naturally when we wake up] close your eyes and take a few deep breaths.

Sense the energy emanating from the skies, bring your arms round to the front at shoulder level and reach up to the skies, imagine the energies between you and the sky and gather it up in your arms, visualising it in whatever form is easy for you.

With your hands, bring the energy into the part of your body that needs a helping hand. The area in the central chest is a great choice, there is a vortex there called 'Heaven Rushing In' and let it do just that.

Hold for however long is comfortable for you – I will often do for a couple of minutes in the morning when I walk the dogs at sunrise or sunset and really feel the transition between day and night, yin and yang.

A great way to activate your Yin/feminine energy for self care and nurturing. It is uplifting when you feel in despair, lonely or at a junction in your life where you just don't know which way to turn. By connecting you invisibly to something greater than you, to a spiritual realm, you realise you are not alone, trust that you are exactly where you should be in your life and all will unfold and be well.

Fabulous figure 8'ing

This is one to do on your own and really let go. Moving your hips and body in figure 8 patterning, stimulates each and every one of your 'Strangeflows' – flows in the body of energy that carry joy and help you cope with change in your life. Great for loosening the hips and back.

Start by raising your arms above your head and circling your hips in one direction, then the other, then imagine you are tracing a figure 8 on the floor, close your eyes and go into your own world, free from inhibitions and dance the 8's flowing easily. Arms can go where they want.

Sumo suspension

Can be done standing or in a chair.

Release the hips, pelvis, shoulders, spine and diaphragm. It activates all major meridian pathways so a great overall general body balancing and so quick and easy. Stimulates cerebral spinal fluid so keeps you alert

- Stand with feet wide apart, certainly wider than the shoulders, feet facing forward.

- Place palms of hands on the thighs just above the knees

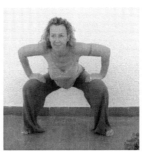

- Put your weight into your hands/knees. Keep your arms straight

- Lean forward and push the knees out with the hands.

- Gently rock from side to side, experiment with your balance.

- When you are ready, bring your left shoulder to your right knee, stretching out the back – stay there for a few seconds

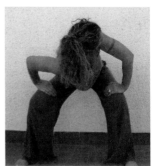

- Come back to the centre and repeat on the other side, right shoulder to left knee.

- Experiment with the positioning of your hands on your thighs – nearer the knee or the groin, what feels good? Fingertips on inner or outer thigh – which way stretches you more?

ENERGY TIPS FOR EVERYDAY LIFE

- Try not to use a shoulder bag as they cut right across crucial energy pathways. If you do use one, do a cross crawl and massage K27 to correct the damage. Remember K27 from the 4 thumps – in the junction of the collar bones and breastbone.

- Try not to wear an under wired bra. Not only do they cut through energy lines, they also sit right on key lymphatic reflexes and can cause congestion of the energy in that vital breast area. If you do wear one, firmly massage the areas where the wire sits, once you have taken the bra off. *Be careful also, I noticed last week a warning on a bra, asking that it is not worn for more than 8 consecutive hours because of the 'elastic' they use, I would be slightly concerned if my bra came with a warning!*

· Try not to sleep surrounded by electrical appliances – make your bedroom an EMF free zone. If you do succumb to a TV, radio alarm clock etc., place a purple amethyst close to them to absorb any of the negative EMFs.

· Shaking hands in greeting. Our traditional handshake originated as an acknowledgement to your opponent, not your friend. You will lose energy. The solution is to use both your hands in the shake. I personally think it is a warmer greeting and it won't weaken you.

· After any aerobic exercise, do a cross crawl. A lot of the movements typical in these classes, such as 'jumping jacks' will drain or flip your energy from a crossing into a homeolateral patterning.

· After working out in the gym always do some simple stretching. It will remove any constriction or congestion in the tissue and make space for energies to move freely.

· Before walking, jogging or running always massage K27 for 15 seconds to ensure you will be moving with your energy, not against it.

· Driving and feeling tired. Especially around your eyes? Pull over, breathe deeply and firmly massage the K27 points for an instant energy shot.

- Feel a cold coming on? Quickly do the 'Connecting Heaven and Earth' or the variation in this booklet. They have the power to nip a cold in the bud, but you have to do it at the very first sign.

- Fallen over, hurt or shocked in any way? Hold the site of the pain and put your other palm against your forehead firmly and breathed deeply for a few minutes. It will reduce the pain.

- Clear clutter from your thoughts, home, office and car. It clears a path for you to move forward.

- Drink lots of water, not just for hydration but also for the health of your internal 'electrical' circuits.

- Reduce stress instantly by placing palm on forehead, close your eyes and breathe.

- Get enough sleep, many of us suffer from sleep deprivation. It is vital for our healing, replenishing for every aspect of our well being.

- Wherever there is pain in the body there will be stagnation and reduced movement of blood, lymph, nerves, energy. Create space for flow and healing. When you have pain, how can you stretch it out? Use your imagination and experiment; the more you work with your energies the more intuitive you will become and you will automatically find the right movements.

- And finally – smile and laugh, as Eric Idle sang at the Olympics: *"Always look on the bright side of life"*

Madison 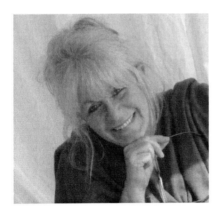 King

Writer & Teacher of Energy Medicine

Madison's Medicine is a unique fusion of energy and body work, flower essences, lifestyle advice and commonsense – providing essential, everyday, practical tools for a healthier and happier you.

Many moons ago Madison was involved in the heart of London advertising, becoming a successful international board director. However, she realised, after a few ambition fuelled years, that she wanted her life to take a different direction and shocked everyone by giving up the BMW, Armani suits and Gucci briefcase, becoming a student again.

She trained in massage, sports massage, aromatherapy, Indian head massage, reflexology, trager, nutrition, flower essences, crystals, radionics... A true workshop groupie, she filled a wall with qualifications but could not find what she had been seeking; she couldn't even really define it... until, through divine synchronicity, she met Donna Eden in London through a mutual friend. Within no time at all she was in Ashland in Donna's backyard with about four other students, eagerly learning about energy – this was more than two decades ago, so no information highway was available in those days and ever the thirsty student she drank in everything she could on these visits, rushing back to London to experiment on her long suffering clients!

Over the years she crossed the ocean many times learning from Donna and also John Thie [Touch for Health].

She then began to teach Donna's work in the UK, USA, Gozo, Malta, Italy, Egypt and many other locations around the world, she has appeared on national television, radio and press promoting EEM. She has lectured at Westminster and Oxford universities and at the key Mind Body Spirit Festivals in London and Wales.

In 2006 she gave up a thriving practice in Central London and now divides her time between the Isle of Wight and the Andalucían town of Nerja in Southern Spain.

Just about to enter her 7th decade, she has set up and is running Donna Eden's training in Europe – based just outside London... a long way from those days in Donna's back yard!

Her focus is on promoting Donna's work in Europe and also writing and teaching her own version: Madison's Medicine, which based on Eden Energy Medicine also weaves in many other natural health threads, giving people simple yet powerful tools to enhance their quality of life on every single level.

As we enter unprecedented waters on this planet, it can be empowering to know that there is always something

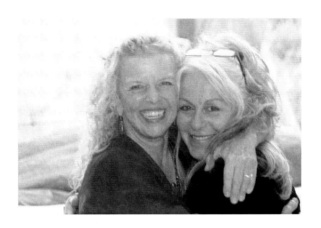

YOU can do to improve any situation, challenge or trauma that life throws into your path.

"Madison is an extraordinary woman and healer. She carries an essence of the highest quality and caring, of camaraderie of spirit, wisdom, compassion and depth of understanding of the healing realms. To train with her is something you will never regret"

Donna Eden – Eden Energy Medicine

Madison can be contacted:

www.madisonking.com
www.midlifegoddess.ning.com
madisonking@hotmail.com

My special thanks to Donna Eden.[8]
*Without her friendship and generous, unselfish
sharing of her vast knowledge, I would not be who I
am today and you would not be reading this book.*

*I also want to thank Alex, Rose and Kleshna for a fun
shoot on the balcony of the Avalon in Nerja – where
we chased the shadows to take the photos that I hope
convey the fun we had and give you a good guide as to
the techniques.*

*A final thanks to Isobel, David and Alex – who have
guided me through wonderful hours of yoga and kept
me sane.*

*www.youtube.com/embed/8zheJRMx4ww to see Isobel
Gilton demonstrating her yoga fusion dance.*

*If you would like to experience the Avalon restaurant
and hostel by the sea in Nerja – visit
www.Avalonnerja.com
Finally, visit Kleshna's site for great jewellery –
www.kleshna.com*

This is meant as a fun guide to energy medicine, if it
whets your appetite for more information on books,
DVD, CDs online study and workshops visit
www.midlifegoddess.ning.com
and also Donna Eden's site , I strongly recommend her
book Energy Medicine
www.innersource.net
You Tube for some great clips
And look out for other books in the Essentials stable

---

8 www.innersource.net